Essential Oils for Migraines

Essential Oil Recipes for **Migraines** for Diffusers, Roller Bottles, Inhalers & more.

Rica V. Gadi

Printed in the United States of America

First Printing, 2019

ISBN: 9781792989902

http://eorecipes.net

DISCLAIMER: This document is a compilation of recipes used successfully by EO enthusiasts who use only high-quality, therapeutic-grade essential oils as determined by many factors including growth, growth location, harvesting process, distillation method used, etc. Please be advised that not all essential oils are created equally, and not all essential oils are suitable for topical use or ingestion. Please do your research before choosing the brand(s) of essential oils you decide to use as well as supplies you use. Always follow label directions on the essential oil bottles.

All the recipes in this book have been inspired by essential oil believers. However, we are not medical practitioners and cannot diagnose, treat or prescribe treatment for any health condition or disease. Just a precaution, before using any alternative medicines, natural supplements, or vitamins, you should always discuss the products you are using or intend to use with your doctor, especially if you are pregnant, trying to get pregnant or nursing.

All information contained within this book is for reference purposes only, and is not intended to substitute advice given by a pharmacist, physician or other licensed health-care professional. As such, the author is not responsible for any loss, claim or damage arising from use of the essential oil recipes contained herein.

This book is dedicated to all the strong people who are taking responsibility of your own well being and doing something to be better.

All my heartfelt gratitude to the following people: my mom Ruby Jane, you have made me everything I am today; my dad Nestor-- my eternal, my angel, and the source of my perseverance; Mommyling, my spiritual guide ; Ria & Joe, the true witnesses of my transformation and my foundation pillars; Ellie Jane, the sparkle of our eyes;

Juan, thanks for always encouraging me to push harder - you are my ONE; Rocco & Radha, my reason for everything.

The Love of my family and friends is the fountain of inspiration that never runs dry. Thank you for constantly inspiring me, motivating me, and loving me unconditionally.

This book will never be complete without the help of my trusted and talented friends the #NOWsuperstars and my #oilbularya friends

Blending Essential Oils to use for a very specific reason has become very popular in the recent years. There are several reasons why this is so. Blending EOs is basically about inhaling - as it has been proven that aromas have the ability to trigger feelings, emotions and personal memories.

With this in mind, it is obvious that everyone is unique when it comes to what triggers your senses. It all boils down to personal preference for the aroma to trigger what you want to unleash. Everyone is different and we all connect to the aroma differently, so what might work for one might not work for another person.

Of course, we also want the blend we personalize to be therapeutic. This is the best reason why to blend essential oils. We want the blend we create to help us with a very specific emotion or physical condition. As much as smelling good is important in a blend, it is more important that we blend oils that is not only pleasing to the smell but also produces the therapeutic effect we are after.

Then you have to think about contraindications. Making sure the blend you create is safe to use.

I suggest that before blending find out if the oils you are using is safe for a condition you may have example, if you are pregnant, or have specific allergies. Consult your physician prior to moving forward.

The recipes I have in this book is a compilation of what has proven to work and favored by hundreds of EO enthusiasts. It takes out the guesswork to get you started.

Again, we urge you to read the recipes and make sure that this is safe for you to try.

The book is very specific to a physical and emotional condition. There are several recipes here because you might want to rotate and you may like one and not the other. There is also a variety of application. Some of us prefer to diffuse, some to make roller bottles, and others to create sprays.

I hope you enjoy this compilation, feel free to use the notes section and jot down your fave blends. There is a wonderful world of EO blending - this is just the beginning.

Rica

A migraine is like a headache that's gone haywire. It is a pulsating, throbbing headache that is normally just on one side of your head.It normally happens with nausea, feelings of or vomiting, annoying sensitivity to noise and light or affects your vision. IT has the ability to stop your from focusing on day-to-day mundane tasks as its pain can last for hours or days and could disable you to function normally.

There is no definite reason as to what causes migraines. Its mysterious source could stem from a disorder in the central nervous system, or a discrepancy in the blood vessel system in your brain or vascular system, it could be your genetic make-up or something with the chemicals in your brain. It's very difficult to pinpoint without further tests.

When a migraine occurs, you may experience one of the following:
Visual Occurrences : the formation of shapes, flashes of light or bright spots, blurring of sight, sensations like poking of needles to the legs or arms, loss of strength on a single side of the body, speech issues, facial numbness, sensitivity to sound, or uncontrollable movements or jerking.

The most common causes of Migraine, according to research, are Stress, Diet and Food Intake and Caffeine Withdrawals or the overconsumption or it.

Migraine usually are not a huge concern. It is however advisable to mention to your health practitioner if you are experiencing one of the following :

- Migraines occur more than 3 times within a week
- Migraines that just gets worse that don't go away
- If your taking a pain med for your migraine everyday or nearly daily for a week
- If you have needed 2 or more doses of OTC pain reliever within a week
- Migraines that affect your daily and social lives

Aromatherapy and essential oils is worth giving a try for migraines for pain relief and management. It may not be a cure for the migraine but has a good potential to help in pain relief or relieve the symptoms that go along with it. Eos have been known to cause tension releasing effects for calming and relaxation or stress reduction to control frequency and the level of severity.

The benefits of Essential Oils for Migraines, when used properly, can aid in relieving your headaches and migraines. It has been known that Eos have the ability to ease the tension that usually contributes or causes many different types of Migraines, not to mention the relaxing and calming effect EOs bring.

Table of Contents

Migraine is defined as a severe headache which usually lasts for three to four days. It can start from only one side of the head but may spread to the other side when time comes. When an episode of migraine attacks you, you may be sensitive to sound and light that might irritate you and ruin your mood, heck even your day. There are a lot of analgesics or painkillers that can be bought in pharmacies and drugstores. However, because of the improvement of medicine up to the modern period, pain killers aren't only in the form of tablets and capsules. Oil or essential oil to be precise is one of the tools that people use in relieving sickness and discomfort nowadays. So we have identified some of the most recommended essential oils for migraine. Please take a read.

Eucalyptus

Eucalyptus is best known for its health-promoting benefits most especially when it comes to mild respiratory ailments such as cough and cold. Due to its antibacterial and antiviral properties, it stops the frequency of cough and gives relief to congestion. But aside from that, it also serves as an effective tool for reducing headaches caused by some respiratory ailments. Most importantly, studies showed that eucalyptus can be an alternative remedy for migraines and headache tension.

How do you use eucalyptus as an essential oil for migraine? You may try to rub a drop or two of the oil onto your chest, this will help in clearing the sinuses which cause headache or migraine when clogged. You may also try to add a few drops of the oil to a pot of hot water and deeply breathe in the vapor.

Lavender

One of the most recognized herb for reducing anxiety and stress due to its sedative properties made it to the list as one of the top recommended remedy for migraine. No wonder why lavender is almost everyone's favorite because it has a lot of uses. In one of the studies, it showed how significant migraine is in combating a migraine attack. The patients suffering from acute migraine attack was partly resolved only by inhaling lavender essential oil.

Lavender essential oil can be used in many ways for treating migraines. Through topical application, apply the diluted lavender essential oil onto your wrists, neck, and bottoms of the feet. As mentioned above, favorable results can be observed in just fifteen minutes through direct inhalation of the oil. You may also add a few drops to your bath to lessen the frequency of migraine attack.

Chamomile

Chamomile has been known for its sedative properties which made it to the list of the most effective essential oils for sleeping. Chamomile is also known for soothing muscle pain and pressure. Not just that, it reduces anxiety and relieves insomnia attack as well which are common causes of headache or migraine. So for this reason, it can be an aid for reducing tension headaches and even migraine. There is an important note for women, however, chamomile must not be used during pregnancy as miscarriage is one of its risk.

During an episode of migraine, you may have a drop of two to a cotton ball and directly inhale. This was proven to reduce the pain and the tension. Through topical application, you may try to rub 2-3 drops of the oil and apply to your wrists, and nape of the neck. The properties and the compound of the essential oil will be absorbed to the bloodstream and will give you a relief from the pain. Lastly, you can use a diffuser or can also add several drops to your bath.

Rosemary

Rosemary is very common to people who often feel nausea and dizziness. However, aside from that, rosemary can also be an effective tool in combating headache tension and migraine attack. Due to its analgesic or pain killing properties, it was proven to have a positive effect on giving relief to the discomfort you feel. Rosemary also reduces anxiety and sleeping problems like anxiety which can be associated with headache or migraine.

To enjoy rosemary benefits, rub a few drops of the oil and massage to the affected area. It can also be applied on to your wrists, nape of the neck, and bottoms of the feet. We suggest you to combine it with a carrier oil like coconut oil for best results. Direct inhalation and using a diffuser can also give you relief from your migraine attack.

Peppermint

This oil is commonly used for respiratory ailments such as cough, cold, sinus congestion and others. Peppermint contains menthol which is effective in relieving muscle pain and tension. So for this reason, peppermint can be used as well to combat headaches and migraines.

Peppermint as an essential oil for migraine can be used through topical application. Rub the oil to to the trigger parts like the base of the skull, nape of the neck, and on your wrists as well. You may also add a few drops of the oil to a glass of hot water and drink the mixture. This is proven to give you relief from the pain caused by migraine.

Headache and migraine can feel so bad that you would even like to knock your head on the door or on a concrete wall. This is the type of discomfort that everyone would not like to experience. However, we can't tell when is it going to attack us so it is better to have an available remedy for this distress. We have listed the benefits of the most recommended essential oils for migraine, so see which one's your favorite. But before you even think of trying, consult your doctor first to know the adverse effects and risks.

It is also worth mentioning that the following oils are worth checking out for Migraines : **Eucalyptus, Sweet Basil, Clary Sage, Rose, Melissa, Jasmine, Spearmint, Helichrysum, Frankincense, Marjoram, Ginger and Neroli**

The Blending Process

These EOs are categorized by aromas, and EOs from the same group usually blend fantastically together.

- Floral – Lavender, Geranium, Jasmine
- Woodsy – Pine, Cedarwood
- Earthy – Vetiver, Patchouli
- Herbaceous – Marjoram, Rosemary, Basil
- Minty – Peppermint, Spearmint, Wintergreen
- Medicinal – Eucalyptus, Frankincense, Melaleuca
- Spicy – Pepper, Clove, Cinnamon
- Oriental – Ginger, Patchouli
- Citrus – Wild Orange, Lemon, Lime

Select oils that will give you with the health benefits you are looking to remedy. For increased energy choose: Grapefruit, Lemon, Orange, or Citrus. For Calming and Relaxation choose: Lavender, Cedarwood, or Chamomile. You are encouraged to experiment and play with your oils to see which blends work for you.

TIPS:

- Combine Floral EOs with Woodsy, Spicy and Citrus aromas
- Minty EOs with Woodsy, Earthy, Herbaceous and Citrus aromas
- Earthy EOs with Woodsy and Minty aromas
- Citrus EOs with Floral, Woodsy, Minty, Spicy and Oriental aromas

Diffuse

Diffusing Essential Oils is the safest
method to enjoy Essential Oils
without the risk of an allergic reaction.

Diffusing Essential Oils
Some Tidbits You Need To Know

Our sense of smell is one of our most powerful senses, and as you have noticed in your own experience that some scents affect your more positively in your minds than others. The body contains over 1,000 receptors for smell—way more receptors than for any of our other senses.

Diffusion Essential Oils means the process vaporizes oils into air by releasing tiny amounts into the air. Inhalation is totally safe and is super low risk. Chances of any EO rising to dangerous levels while diffusion is slim to none.

Diffusing Essential Oils around newborns, babies, young children, pregnant or nursing women, and pets should be done with caution. Read up on safety.

It is advisable that Diffusing Essential Oils for only about 15-30 minutes at a time to be most effective. NEVER leave your diffuser on overnight. Make sure your diffuser is filled with the right amount of water and you understand the operating directions.

While diffusing essential oils, be sure that your space has great ventilation. Crack a window open if the scent become to strong.

Never add Carrier Oils to your diffuser. This may cause your diffuser to malfunction. Clean your diffuser at least 3 times a week with warm water and natural soap to ensure the diffuser is well maintained and bacteria and mold does not accumulate.

Diffusing Essential Oils
Basic Guidelines

Just a few things you need to know and prepare before getting started Diffusing Essential Oils.

Things you need:
Ultrasonic Oil Diffuser
Essential Oils
Water

Just follow the number of drops in the recipe, drop on to an oil diffuser and fill the rest with water.

All diffusers are different and will have its own water minimum and maximum level. Read the diffuser instruction before use.

Ideally, it is best to diffuse for 15-30 minutes and turn off the diffuser. The effect should be good for at least 2-3 hours. Turn your diffuser back on after 3 hours to reinforce oil diffusing effects.

It is not advisable to use EO in humidifiers.These are not made to release EOS

Diffuser Recipes

Here's a thought for you:

You may be wondering how aroma can simply eliminate symptoms. There's a simple answer to this : Aroma is simply a by-product of diffusing. It's the added benefit but in reality the real benefit comes from the air we breathe and how the body easily absorbs the essential oils released in the air. It works 2 ways, not only does it improve the air quality you breath by disinfecting and eliminating pollutants it also allows your glands to absorb the healing elements of the EOs released in the air molecules,

So for here are a few recipes that can help you manage symptoms and actual issues regarding the matter :

2 Drops Marjoram
2 Drops Thyme
2 Drops Rosemary
2 Drops Peppermint
2 Drops Lavender"

----

2 Drops Peppermint
2 Drops Lavender
1 Drop Eucalyptus
1 Drop Rosemary

----

4 Drops Lavender
4 Drops Peppermint
2 Drops Frankincense
2 Drops Basil

2 Drops Lavender
2 Drops Wild Orange
1 Drop Geranium
1 Drop Clary Sage

----

3 Drops Peppermint
2 Drops Eucalyptus
1 Drops Myrrh

----

3 Drops Frankincense
3 Drops Lavender
3 Drops Bergamot

----

2 Drops Rosemary
2 Drops Peppermint
2 Drops Lavender

----

5 Drops Clove Bud
2 Drops Frankincense
2 Drops Lemon

----

5 Drops Lavender
3 Drops Lemongrass
2 Drops Peppermint

----

3 Drops Coriander
3 Drops Peppermint
3 Drops Rosemary

3 Drops Lavender
2 Drops Cedarwood
2 Drops Vetiver

----

3 Drops Lavender
3 Drops Geranium
2 Drops Roman Chamomile
2 Drops Clary Sage
2 Drops Ylang Ylang

----

3 Drops Lavender
3 Drops Lime
3 Drops Mandarin

----

4 Drops Lavender
2 Drops Cedarwood
2 Drops Wild Orange
1 Drop Ylang Ylang

----

3 Drops Frankincense
2 Drops Copaiba

----

3 Drops Lavender
2 Drops Stress Away
2 Drops Frankincense

----

5 Drops Frankincense
5 Drops Stress Away

----

3 Drops Peppermint
5 Drops Lavender
2 Drops Stress Away

----

4 Drops Bergamont
5 Drops Frankincense

----

4 Drops Stress Away
4 Drops Orange

----

2 Drops Purification
3 Drops Lemon
3 Drops Orange

----

2 Drops Grapefruit
2 Drops Bergamot
2 Drops Lime
2 Drops Ginger
1 Drop Sandalwood

----

3 Drops Orange
3 Drops Patchouli

----

2 Drops Lavender
2 Drops Cedarwood
2 Drops Roman Chamomile

----

4 Drops Lavender
3 Drops Geranium
2 Drops Roman Chamomile
2 Drops Clary Sage
2 Drops Ylang Ylang

Roll

Essential Oil Roller Bottles is the easiest method to enjoy Essential Oils Anywhere and Whenever.

Essential Oils are usually super concentrated and too hard to measure how much to actually put straight from the bottle.

Roller bottles are a way that you are able to create blends ready to use with the right dilution. It allows your EO to last longer.

It also makes it easier to apply exactly where you want to target without getting it all over the place.

It is handy and easy to carry in your purse, ready to use at any time you want to.

I like to apply EOs at the bottom of the feet for many reasons. Our feet have bigger pores than any other skin in our bodies. this means that they are able to suck in the therapeutic compounds in our blend into the bloodstream faster that any other parts of the body. Imagine comparing a normal straw to an oversized straw and how much more you can suck in with the latter. This is how the soles of our feet is compared to the rest of the skin in our bodies.

The skin on our feet is also less sensitive and is designed to withstand some abuse. The risk of having an irritation from EOS is less likely to happen when applied on the feet.

The feet don't have the glands that act as a barrier. Sebaceous glands are glands in our skin that produces an oily substance called Sebum, for the purpose of lubricating and waterproofing the skin. Since this is oil and if you put oil on top of oil, it can act as a barrier or it may slow down penetration.

The feet and palms of our hands are the only skin that don't have these, so it is ideal to apply Essential Oils to the feet for maximum penetration.

Now, it would be hard to apply oils directly and very mess, right? Roller bottles make it super easy and convenient to roll the EOs at the bottom of our feet.

Carrier Oils Info

Carrier oils are vegetable-based oils with their own healing properties that dilute essential oils used to help carry the EOs into the skin.

Essential oils are highly concentrated and could evaporate very quickly. The carrier oil is mixed with the essential oil so it could penetrate the skin before it actually evaporates. Although EOs are oils, it is actually not that oily. When mixed with a carrier oil, it allows you to have more of the essential oil into your skin without wasting EOS to evaporate, making the healing properties of the EO strong and more effective.

There are also Essential oils that are too strong to apply directly to the skin and may cause damage, so it is important to dilute them with a carrier oil.

Never add Carrier Oils to your diffuser. This may cause your diffuser to malfunction. Clean your diffuser at least 3 times a week with warm water and natural soap to ensure the diffuser is well maintained and bacteria and mold does not accumulate.

Carrier Oils

There are a lot of different carrier oils that you can use with EOs to dilute them in a roller bottle.

To name a few :

Almond Oil - moisturizing and stays liquid at room temperature. Do not use if you are allergic to nuts.

Apricot Kernel Oil - moisturizing and suitable for sensitive skin or kids. It is super gentle on the skin.

Avocado Oil - moisturizing and suitable for sensitive and damaged skin. Perfect for skin problems.Can be mixed with other carrier oils

Castor Oil - with antibacterial, antiviral and antifungal properties, use topically to eliminate pain and relieve skin irritation.

Coconut Oil - its antibacterial, antiviral and antifungal properties it is the best and most versatile for skin care. The skin absorbs this very quickly. It solidifies in room temp and may still have a slight coconut oil aroma in it - but you can get a fractionated coconut oil to eliminate the 2 challenges above.

Grapeseed Oil - not just for cooking but also great for topical application on the skin.

Jojoba Oil - one of my faves for skin care blends. This oil is the closest to our natural oil our skin produces to it is absorbed easily without being oily. Also amazing for massage oil blends.

Olive Oil - this is the oil for herb type oils. mostly used for cooking but can also be applied to the skin but would need to be blended with a carrier oil that is mild and absorb well with the skin.

Rosehip Seed Oil - super good for deep moisturizing or skin irritations. This oil has a high content of antioxidants and helps remedy dry, scarred and wounded skin.

Recommended Roller Bottle Dilution Guide

RECOMMENDED ROLL-ON BOTTLE DILUTION AMOUNTS

5 ml (1/6 oz.) Roll-on Bottle = ~100 drops (1tsp.)
10 ml (1/3 oz.) Roll-on Bottle = ~200 drops (2 tsp.)
30 ml. (1 oz.) Roll-on Bottle = ~600 drops (6 tsp.)

Roll-on Size	5 ml	10 ml	30 ml	Add EO drops to roll-on, then fill with carrier oil.	
Essential Oil Drops	1	2	6	1%	Dilution Percentage
	2	4	12	2%	
	3	6	18	3%	
	5	10	30	5%	
	10	20	60	10%	
	20	40	120	20%	
	25	50	150	25%	
	50	100	300	50%	

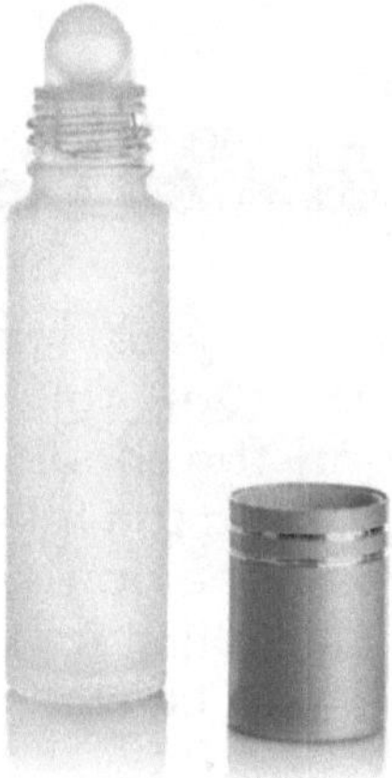

General Guidelines:
Birth to 12 months = .3-.5% dilution
1-5 years = 1.5-3% dilution
6-11 years = 1.5-5% dilution
12-17 years = 1.5-20% dilution
18 years and older = 1.5% dilution-Neat (no dilution)
Elderly or Sensitive Skin = 1-3% dilution
Daily Use = 2-5% dilution
Short Term Use = 10-25% dilution
Local Skin or Systemic Issues = 50% dilution-Neat

These are general guidelines suggestions--not absolute rules--based on traditional aromatheraphy practice. (Kurt Schnaubelt PhD, Valerie Worwood, Robert Tisserand)

Dilution Basics:

How much you dilute your EO depends on different factors such as weight, sensitivity, health conditions, EOs that are blended in or how long that blend has been used for. There is never an absolute dilution rule, it is you who knows about your level and tolerance. I feel that it is best to start with a higher dilution percentage and increase EO drops over time.

To make sure your EO is safe, make sure that the oils you use are therapeutic grade and do your research on the source and extraction methods used to produce the oils.

Roller Bottle Blending Order

I normally just start with dropping the drops of oils into the **10mL roller bottle**, then adding the carrier oil up until the shoulder of the bottle. Capping the bottle off with the roller and the bottle cap. Instead of shaking the bottle, i like to roll the bottle between my palms first for a minute or 2 for blending, then finishing it off with a few shakes.

NOTE: All recipes in this book is for a 10mL Roller Bottle. If you have a bigger or smaller roller bottle, adjust the number of EO drops based on the size of your bottle.

Roller Bottle Recipes

2 drops Copaiba
2 drops Peppermint
2 drops Wintergreen
2 drops Marjoram
3 drops Lavender
3 drops Eucalyptus Globolus

----

3 drops Peppermint
2 drops Clove
3 drops Wintergreen
2 drops Ginger

----

4 drops Lavender
4 drops Frankincense
4 drops Copaiba
4 drops Peppermint

----

4 drops Peppermint
4 drops Frankincense
4 drops Lavender

----

4 drops Peppermint
2 drops Frankincense
2 drops Lavender
2 drops Chamomile

----

4 drops PanAway
4 drops Valor
3 drops Copaiba
3 drops Peppermint

----

3 drops Frankincense
2 drops Lavender
2 drops Sacred Mountain
2 drops Valor
2 drops Royal Hawaiian Sandalwood

----

3 drops Peppermint
2 drops Basil
2 drops Lemongrass
3 drops Frankincense

----

2 drops Frankincense
2 drops Lavender
4 drops Cypress
1 drop Ginger
1 drop Peppermint

----

4 drops Lavender
4 drops Peppermint
2 drops Frankincense

----

5 drops Lavender
3 drops Peppermint
2 drops Eucalyptus

----

4 drops Frankincense
4 drops Lavender
4 drops Peppermint

----

5 drops Bergamot
5 drops Frankincense

----

3 drops Stress Away
2 drops Lavender
2 drops Frankincense
2 drops Patchouli
1 drops Valor
1 drops White Angelica

----

7 drops Eucalyptus Radiata
5 drops Rosemary
3 drops Grapefruit

----

4 drops Frankincense
3 drops Bergamot
2 drops Orange
2 drops Grapefruit
2 drops Clary Sage

----

5 drops Eucalyptus
5 drops Spearmint

----

3 drops Lavender
3 drops Valor
2 drops Vetiver
2 drops Grapefruit
2 drops Joy
1 drops Release
1 drops Cedarwood

Bonus Recipes

Pain Relief Massage Oil Favorite

60mL Jojoba Oil (cold pressed)
8 drops Lavender
8 drops Peppermint
15 drops Frankincense

Pain Relief Massage Oil Secret

14 drops Frankincense
10 drops Sweet Orange
8 drops Turmeric
30mL Sweet Almond Oil

Pain Relief Bath Soak Blend

10 drops Frankincense
5 drops Lavender
5 drops Bergamot
1 cup Full-Cream/ Full-Fat Milk

Pain Relief Bath Salt Blend

1 cup Epsom Salt
¼ cup Dead Sea Salt
¼ cup Baking Soda
8-10 drops Essential Oils
(use any ingredient above or single oils)

Inhale

Essential Oil Inhalers are the most convenient way to enjoy Essential Oils Anywhere and Whenever.

Essential Oil Inhalers give you quick and easy access to the vast therapeutic benefits of essential oils.

Blending Essential Oils in an Inhaler
Some Tidbits You Need To Know

EO Inhalers or aroma sticks are compact tubes, with a cotton wick inside and a protective cover, to lock the aroma within.

Your preferred blend of essential oils is absorbed by the cotton wick, and safely enclosed in a tube that that fits inside of the cover. The cover is easily removed for access to the tube to breathe in the aroma. Usually lasts about 3 months, depending on the oil blend used.

I absolutely love these because they encourage me to take a moment during super stressful moments, and just breathe.

It is in times of stress when our breathing patterns often change and taking deep breaths promote a feeling of calm and inner peace. Breath work combined with visualization plus a relaxing inhaler, can offer relief to symptoms of stress and help your body to come back to the state of homeostasis.

Aroma Sticks can be carried in your tiny purse, even compact enough to fit in your pocket. You can enjoy your favorite EOs anywhere and you can use them with discretion.

I love diffusing, and do all the time but not everyone in my space may enjoy the scents I enjoy or they may not benefit from the therapeutic benefits of the EOs I am diffusing - so the inhaler is one way to not only enjoy my choice of blends but to keep in personal not affecting everyone else around me.

Inhalers not only benefits me but also keep those around me safe in case the oils I want to blend may pose a risk to those around me who may have health issue not advised to be exposed to my choice EOs/

When making Aroma Sticks, You may use your chosen EOs at 100% Concentration.

Inhaler Basic Guidelines

Breathe in slow and deep to absorb the EO molecules directly into your olfactory system.

Inhalers are super easy to use. You just remove the cap and inhale from the inhaler tube, count 1 to 5 slowly as you inhale. The EO molecules get drawn into our bloodstream through our nasal cavity and gets delivered throughout our entire body.

Simple to use, easy to cary, portable and compact. You never have to be without your favorite blends, ever.

Inhaler Blending Basics

Inhalers are super easy and simple to make.

All you need is an inhaler set which consist of the following:

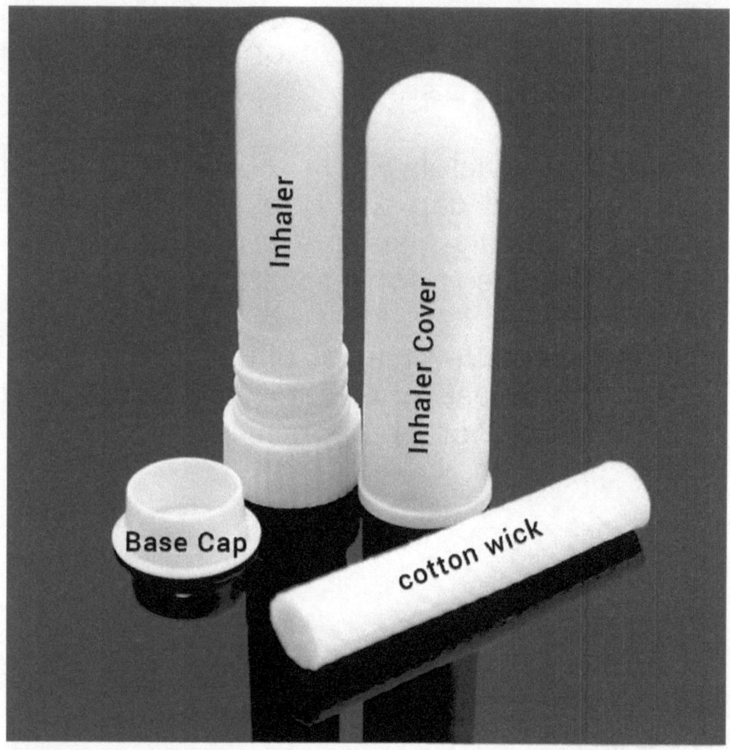

Inhaler, Inhaler Cover, Base Cap and Cotton Wick.

You will need your Essential Oils.

I like to use a pipette for precision and a small petri dish so I can see the oil.

Blending is super easy, just combine the drops and swirl it around in the petri dish and when you are satisfied you can go ahead and drop the cotton wick to absorb all the oil in the dish.

Once the wick is ready you can drop it in the inhaler and cap the bottom with the Base Cap. I usually like to secure the cover with the inhaler so I don't have to do it later.

I usually us 15-20 drops of EO total in a recipe and it can last up to 3 months. Some recipes will need more but on average it is in this range.

Inhaler Recipes

2 Drops of Chamomile
6 Drops of Cedarwood or Sandalwood
3 Drops of Geranium
3 Drops of Bergamot
4 Drops of Lavender

----

10 drops of Roman Chamomile
5 drops of Lavender
3 drops of Vetiver

----

10 drops of Palmarosa
5 drops of Geranium
5 drops of Lavender

----

4 drops Lavender
4 drops Orange
4 drops Frankincense
3 drops Cedarwood

----

6 drops Lavender
5 drops Lime
4 drops Spearmint

----

8 drops of Lavender
4 drops of Roman Chamomile

----

8 drops of Roman Chamomile
8 drops of Lavender
6 drops of Majoram
1 drop of Vetiver

----

8 drops of M-Grain
4 drop of Peppermint

----

6 drops of Peppermint
3 drops of Frankincense
3 drops of Lavender
3 drops of Chamomile

----

10 drops of Geranium
3 drops of Eucalyptus
3 drops of Grapefruit
3 drops of Lavender

----

5 drops of Stress Away
5 drops of Lavender

----

4 drop of Lavender
4 drop of Roman Chamomile
4 drop of Orange

----

5 drops of Bergamot
4 drops of Orange
3 drops of Lemon
3 drops of Grapefruit

----

5 drops of Spruce
4 drops of Cedarwood
3 drops of Juniper
3 drops of White Fir

----

10 drops of Vetiver
6 drops of Sandalwood
5 drops of Geranium

----

10 drops of Orange
5 drops of Clary Sage
5 drops of Ginger

----

4 drops of Grapefruit
3 drops of Spruce
3 drops of Geranium
1 drop of Palmarosa

----

10 drops of Ylang Ylang
6 drops of Lavender
4 drops of Patchouli

----

12 drops of Bergamot
6 drops of Lavender
2 drops of Frankincense

----

6 drops of Sweet Orange
5 drops of Frankincense
4 drops of Clary Sage

<u>Book Ordering</u>

To order your copy / copies of

Essential Oils
for Migraines

please visit: **EOrecipes.net**

You can also check out other titles available.

Bulk Pricing and
Affiliate Programs Available